Health Benefits of Thyme

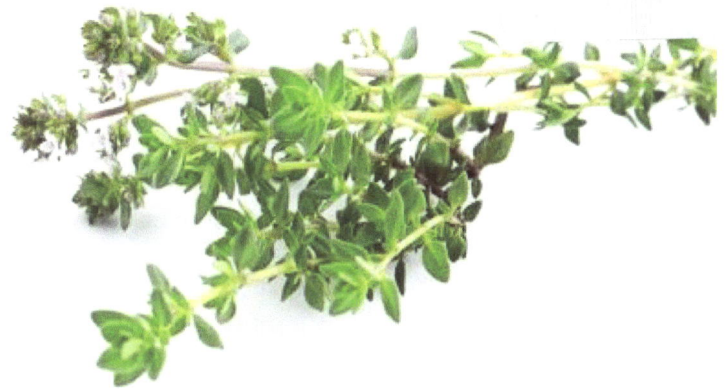

For Cooking and Health

By M. Usman

Health Learning Series

Mendon Cottage Books

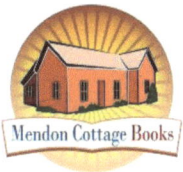

JD-Biz Publishing

Download Free Books!

http://MendonCottageBooks.com

Disclaimer

The information is this book is provided for informational purposes only. It is not intended to be used and medical advice or a substitute for proper medical treatment by a qualified health care provider. The information is believed to be accurate as presented based on research by the author.

The contents have not been evaluated by the U.S. Food and Drug Administration or any other Government or Health Organization and the contents in this book are not to be used to treat cure or prevent disease or mental illness.

The author or publisher is not responsible for the use or safety of any diet, procedure or treatment mentioned in this book. The author or publisher is not responsible for errors or omissions that may exist.

Warning

The Book is for informational purposes only and before taking on any diet, treatment or medical procedure it is recommended to consult with your primary care provider.

Our books are available at

1. Amazon.com
2. Barnes and Noble
3. Itunes
4. Kobo
5. Smashwords
6. Google Play Books

Table of Contents

Getting Started

Chapter # 1: Intro

Thyme itself is not a plant or an herb; it is a collective name given to any one of the many flowering shrubs of the Thymus genus. Thyme is a member of the mint family and is a bushy, wood-based shrub with small yet highly fragranced, grayish green leaves followed by bands of pink or purple colored flowers in the early summers; it grows 15 – 30 cm tall and can be 40 cm wide. There are more than 350 different varieties of thyme all over the world, with French thyme or thymus vulgaris and lemon thyme being the most popular ones; further varieties are stated in the next chapters. Although there are a great many numbers of varieties, the general characteristics of each thyme are usually the same and it is only the color and dimensions that varies.In the medical community, the different species of thymes are distinguished by the composition of their essential oils.

Thyme is incredibly versatile and blends seamlessly with almost all kinds of foods, especially in combination with basil, lemon and garlic.Generally, thyme enlightens and brings up the flavor of any dish. This is the reason as to why many of the Italian and French recipes incorporate thyme in their ingredient list. In addition to its culinary benefits, thyme is also used in aromatherapy.

The essential oils of thyme are used in many traditional as well as clinical medicines due to their anti-viral, anti-septic, anti-parasitic, anti-rheumatic and anti-fungal properties. To delve a little deeper, thyme is a very strong detoxifying agent making it an ingredient in many of the detox food items. The herb is an excellent immunity booster, encourages white blood formation and resistance to harmful organisms. Thyme is also very effective against infections, digestive and respiratory to highlight a few. It can be taken as a cure to diarrhea and infections in the vagina (including thrush) & fallopian tubes. Its power as an anti-septic can be understood from the fact that as less as 1% thyme oil can be used to make a solution to treat gum and mouth infections. In addition, thyme is also a used as relaxant due to its soothing effect on the bronchi muscles; it helps to relieve recurring cough, asthma, dry coughs, laryngitis and bronchitis. Last but not the least, thyme being a digestive herb enhances appetite, digestion and stimulation of the liver. This is the extent of the medical properties the introduction will go to; detailed accounts on the medicinal properties of thyme will be given in subsequent sections.

Thyme is considered native to Asia and southern Europe, i.e. Mediterranean basin; it has also been cultivated in Northern America and is known to thrive there as well.

According to the Georgetown University Medical Center, the prevalence of thyme as a medically viable herb can be traced as back as 460 BC when Hippocrates, also known as the father of Western Medicine recognized it and documented its benefits in his work, Hippocratic Corpus. This is why most of the civilizations on the banks of the Mediterranean were prosperous and long-lasting. Some of these include:

• The Ancient Egyptians had found use of it and were mummifying the corpses of their pharaohs with it.

• The Ancient Greeks used it to burn incense in their temples and in their baths; they believed of it as a source of courage.

• Romans used it to purify their rooms and to give aromatic flavoring to alcoholic beverage and cheese.

During the middle Ages, when folklores were at their peak, people placed thyme beneath their pillows to ward-off nightmares. Thyme leaves were also given by women to their knights and warriors as a good luck charm and to increase their valor. Thyme was also used in pre-medicinal era bandages to treat infections. Prior to the invention of artificial refrigerants, thyme was used to preserve meats and other food products.

It is quite evident that the benefits of thyme are unending and were respected by every civilization so keep on reading if you don't want to miss out on these amazing doles.

Chapter # 2: Nutritional Worth

Thyme is known to contain several active principles that have a disease preventing& boosting effect on the body. Thyme contains the essential oil thymol as well as flavanoid antioxidants that are necessary for the body to keep up its functions. Moreover, it is packed with vitamins and minerals needed for optimum health. The leaves of the thyme plant are some of the most concentrated sources of potassium, manganese, calcium, iron, selenium and magnesium.

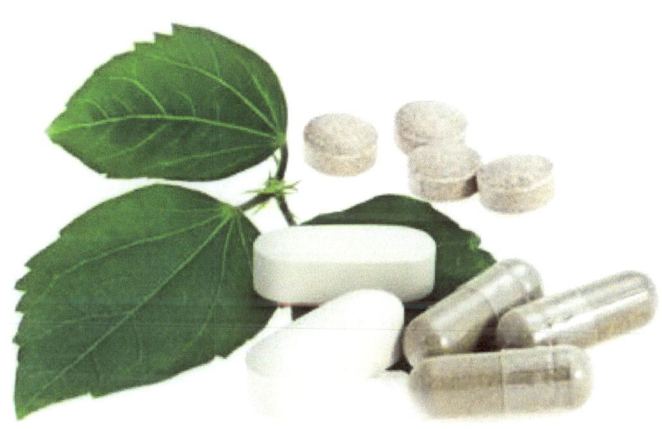

In a nutshell, with respect to the body's daily need a 100 g dose of fresh thyme leaves contain:

i.   38% of dietary fiber

ii.   27% of vitamin B-6

iii.   40% of calcium

iv.   40% of magnesium

v.   75% of manganese

vi.   158% of vitamin A

vii.   218% of iron

viii.   266% of vitamin C

ix.   No cholesterol!

A detailed account of the nutritional wellness of thyme is given in the following tables.

The following chart shows the principle nutritional facts per 100 grams serving of thyme:

Basic Macronutrients & Calories

Nutrient	Amount	Percentage RDA
Energy	101 Kcal	5%
Carbohydrates	24.45 g	18%
Protein	5.56 g	10%
Total Fat	1.68 g	8.4%
Cholesterol	0 mg	0%
Dietary Fiber	14.0 g	37%

The next chart shows the details of the vitamins in a 100 grams serving of thyme:

Vitamins

Nutrient	Amount	Percentage RDA
Folates	45 mmg	11%
Niacin	1.824 mg	11%
Pantothenic acid	0.409 mg	8%
Pyridoxine	0.348 mg	27%
Riboflavin	0.471 mg	36%
Thiamin	0.48 mg	4%
Vitamin A	4751 IU	158%
Vitamin C	160.1 mg	266%

The final chart shows the electrolytes and minerals stuffed in a 100 grams serving of thyme.

Minerals

Nutrient	Amount	Percentage RDA
Sodium	9 mg	0.5%
Potassium	609 mg	13%
Calcium	405 mg	40.5%
Iron	17.45 mg	218 %
Magnesium	160 mg	40%
Manganese	1.719 mg	75%
Zinc	1.81 mg	16.5%

Chapter # 3: Selection and Storage

Fresh, dried and powdered; every form of thyme is readily available in the market, all year long. But the question is not of quantity but that of quality; always prioritize fresh thyme over the dried form since it is more flavorful and contains more nutrients compared to dried thyme; the storage life for already dried leaves is about a week. Fresh thyme is sold in bunches of sprigs; a spring is defined as a single stem that has been snapped from the plant. The stem is of woody appearance and is laced with flowers & leaves. The leaves of the fresh thyme you choose should be lively, of vibrant green-gray color and be devoid of any yellow or dark spots. With dried thyme, try to choose the herb that is organically grown, giving it a greater chance of not being irradiated. If you are fortunate enough to have your own thyme plant in the garden (which you will be able to do after reading the next chapter!), pick the thyme leaves as soon as the flowers start to appear as the leaves are the sweetest at that time.

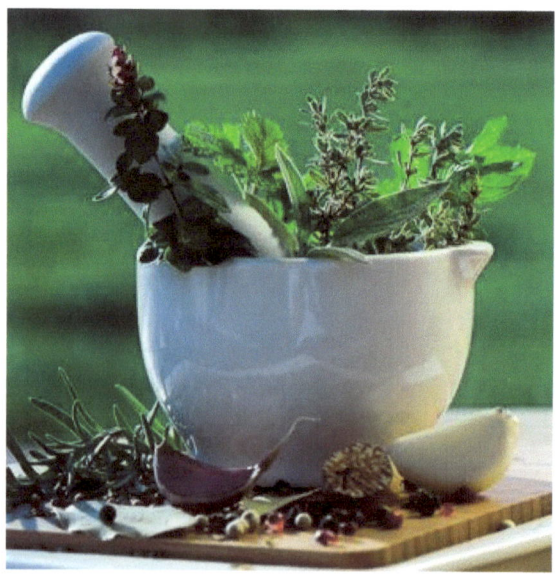

No doubt that dried herbs and spices like thyme are readily available in supermarkets and grocery stores, it is still better if you are able to find a dedicated spice store in your vicinity. The reason for this is simple; as these stores are selective in what they sell, they have a more expansive and higher-grade selection of herbs & spices that those of regular supermarkets.

After fresh thyme has been purchased, it should be refrigerated in a slightly wet paper towel enclosure. Dried thyme is best stored in a tightly sealed glass, kept in a dark, cool and dry place which can increase its freshness to about 6 months. When making dishes with fresh thyme, remember that one fresh sprig of thyme equals half a tablespoon of the dried variant.

To make your own dried version of thyme, hang bundles of thyme sprigs upside down in a dry, warm and airy location for a period of 10 days. After that crush them using your hands and store them as instructed. Also if you are adding thyme leaves directly to your recipe, it is best to remove the stem with the help of a fork as it can be woody and rather annoying.

Chapter # 4: Growing Thyme

This process can be best explained in the form of steps that are as follows:

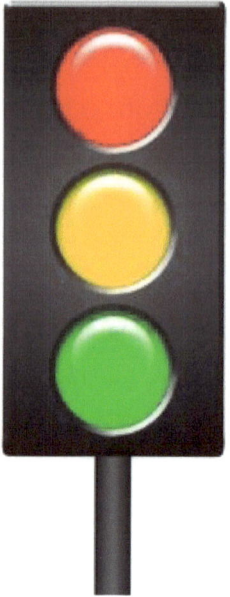

1. **Visit a nursery and acquire thyme plant seedlings:**

Thyme is a quite diverse plant and gives you quite a lot of options when it comes to its growth: it can be grown using plant divisions, seeds, and seedlings; indoor or outdoor. Still, it takes about 1 year for a thyme plant to grow so the easiest method is to purchase seedlings.

2. **Search for a perfect spot to plant the seedlings:**

It's best to grow thyme in full sun and well-drained soil. If the soil appears to be wet then add some sand, compost or organic material to improve the drainage. In addition, thyme can also be planted around paving stones, near a wall or as a ground cover.

3.   As soon as the ground feels warm, plant the seedlings.

4.   While planting the seedlings, make sure to leave 8 – 12 inches of space between them.

Removing weeds around your newly planted herb is an important step and should be carried out on a regular basis.

5.   Harvest the thyme:

Thyme usually grown 6 – 12 inches long, but this is not the major indictor of the time to initiate harvesting. When the plants begin to flower, cut off the first half of the plant; if you want dry thyme then leave it to dry otherwise use it as per your wish. Harvest thyme during the summers but do not do so during fall as it limits the chances of the plant growing back again.

Chapter # 5: Species of Thyme

There is an ever increasing amount of thyme collectors in the world; they are aware of thyme's health & culinary benefits and therefore make the most of their time collecting and planting different species of thyme. You just might be one of them someday so here are some of the most popular species of thyme:

1. **Archer's Gold Thyme** – It is thyme of lemony scents which is of golden color during the winter but during the summer turns bright green.

Height: 6 – 8 inches.

2. **Bressingham Thyme** – It is a trailing type of thyme that develops starry pink colored flowers. It is mostly used for decorations and for its scent.

Height: 3 inches

3. **Caraway Thyme**–Caraway earns its name due to its rich flavor; it is incorporated in dishes such as breads and beef cuts.

Height: 4-8 inches

4. **Doone Valley Thyme** – Leaves are initially of dark green color with specks of gold that turns solid green due to summer's heat and becomes reddish during the winter. It is a trailing type and has a lemon scent.

Height: 2 – 4 inches

5. **English Thyme** – It is very nutritious specie of thyme and has been in use by Europeans since ancient times. It is used in Italian meat dishes and to cover rock gardens.

Height: 12 – 18 inches

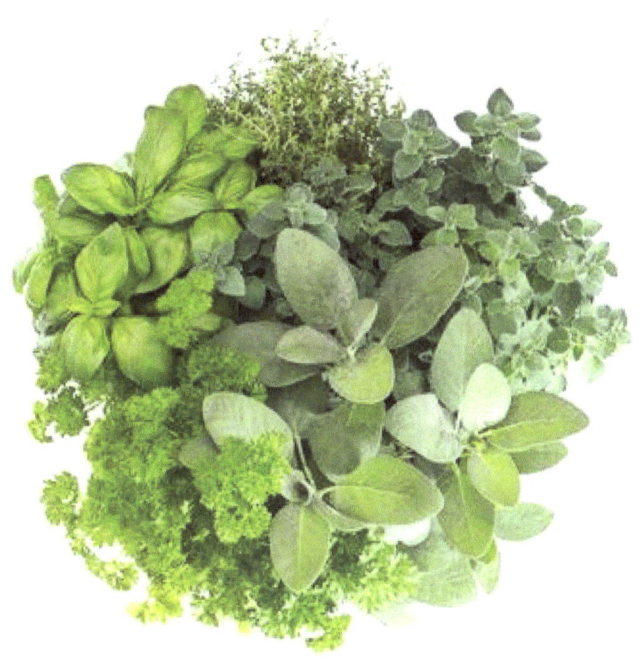

6. **French Thyme** – Considered the top ranked thyme with respect to both culinary and medicinal properties, the French thyme originates from the Mediterranean and has been used in breads, butters and vinegars.

Height: 12 – 18 inches

7. **Golden Thyme** – Consists of green & gold colored leaves and usually grows in a mounding dome.

Height: 6 – 12 inches

8. **Lemon Thyme** – As the name implies, the lemon thyme has a lemon scent and is also an excellent addition in salads, fish and poultry.

Height: 2 – 6 inches

9. **Minus Thyme**–If looked upon closely, appears to be a moss. The minus thyme has very tiny leaves that are extremely dense; it is very aromatic and ornamental nonetheless.

Height: 1 – 2 inches

10. **Wedgewood Thyme**– Considered one of the most ornamental specie in the whole thyme family, Wedgewood thyme has beautiful dark colored foliage with bands of chartreuse and inconsistent growth.

Height: 12 – 18 inches.

Health Benefits of Thyme

Chapter # 6: Intro

The health promoting benefits of thyme are linked to its essential oil, referred to as "oil of thyme"; it packs 20 – 54% thymol that is a natural occurring chemical having the ability to fight and annihilate life-threatening organisms like microbes. Thyme is best known for its cures for respiratory & chest problems that include bronchitis, coughs & chest congestion. However, in recent times researchers have uncovered the curtain on many other components in the oil of thyme making it a candidate against more than just lung diseases. Read and find out.

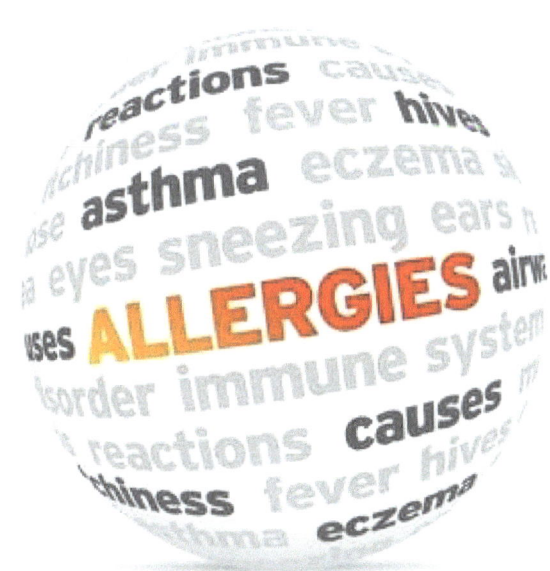

Chapter # 7: Acne

This might seem like something of little importance and relevance, but for some people this particular feature can be a make or break deal. In today's world where perfection is looked-out for the most, things as small as acne can matter the most to some people and it is exactly this fact that several pharmaceutical companies are cashing out on.

Acne is a skin disease related to the oil glands at the base of the hair follicles; these glands get activated during puberty due to hormones produced by adrenal glands. It is not a life threatening issue but still can be something of a pickle for some people. A person suffers from acne when the follicles get blocked, resulting in the build-up of oil; this build-up then results in what are called pimples.

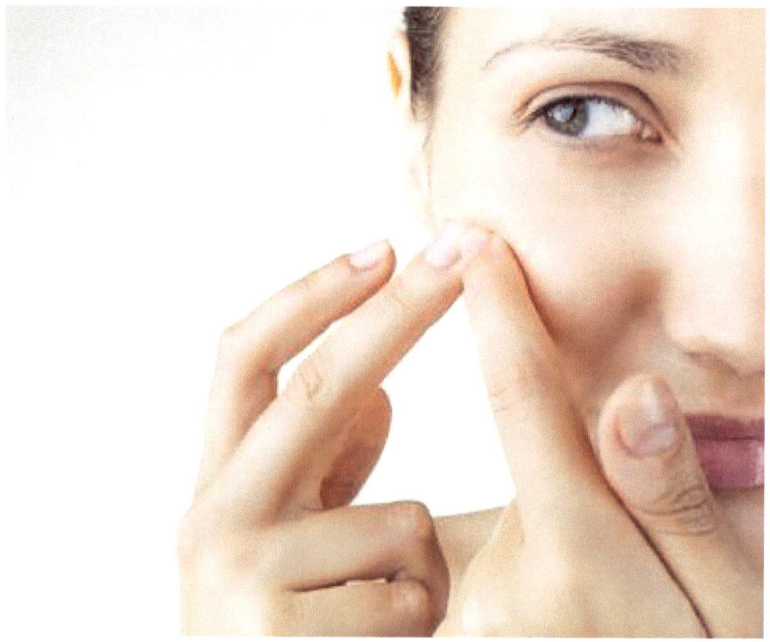

There are many cures for pimples, most popular of them being prescription creams; but according to a research presented by the Leeds Metropolitan University at the Society for General Microbiology's Spring Conference in Dublin, thyme preparations were able to provide a more effective way in treating acne. The researchers from Leeds Metropolitan University tested the healing effects of different tinctures including marigold, myrrh and thyme. The subject of their study was Propionibacterium acne that is the bacteria known for causing acne by infecting pores in the skin and forming spots that can range from simple white heads to puss-filled cysts. During the tests the group found out that while each of the tincture was able to eliminate the bacteria after a time period of 5 minutes, thyme proved to be the most effective one. The group further discovered that the tincture of thyme had an even greater anti-bacterial effect than the standard active ingredient in anti-acne creams: benzyl chloride. This was the first study of its kind, which compared the effects of tinctures on a class of bacteria that caused acne.

The tincture of each of the plant was made by steeping every sample in alcohol for 2 – 3 weeks. This was done to extract the active compounds of the plant. The researchers then used a standard model known as vitro model to test and compare the effects of variable substances applied to the skin. Finally, the effects of the tinctures were compared against an alcohol control to confirm that the anti-bacterial effect was not just due to sterilization of the bacteria.

Still, scientists advice that one should not just start rubbing the essential oil of thyme all over his/her face, the next time a zit pops up. A tried and tested way to make a thyme-inspired cream is given below:

For this treatment, a total of two things are required:

i.   Dried Thyme

ii.   Witch Hazel

Follow the following steps to create a thyme/witch hazel infusion:

i.   Take a small bottle or jar and sterilize it by boiling it in water for about 10 minutes.

ii.   Add one tablespoon of dried thyme to the bottle.

iii.   Pour 4 tablespoons of witch hazel over it.

iv.   Shake the mixture well.

v.   Within about 20 minutes, the witch hazel would appear like a light brown colored tea. If this is what you see, then you have successfully executed the steps up till now.

vi.   Leave the mixture and let the thyme steep in the witch hazel for a few days after which you are free to strain the thyme out.

vii.   Store the infusion in a cool and dark place; it will be usable for a month.

Use this toner, once a day; if you are really concerned about your appearance, there is no harm in using it twice a day. The procedure is simple; pour it on a cotton cloth or a facial pad and swipe it over your face.

The importance of thyme as a natural dermatological fighter may be undermined in developed countries but it should be known that this particular cure is considered a natural gift in the more poorer areas of the world where plant derived medicines are the only choice people have. A research team at the All African Leprosy and Dermatology Education and Training Center at the Addis Abada University carried out randomized, double-blind and placebo-controlled trial to study the effectiveness of thyme oil along with chamomile against common dermatological problems. A 3% thyme oil extract along with 10% chamomile extract was made into a cream to treat eczema-like abrasions. A total of 14 people were subjected to this test; ten subjects were treated with the custom made cream while four were kept on a placebo treatment. The group treated with thyme activated cream completely healed with no adverse effects. This showed that only a 3% thyme oil concentration solution can be used as an inexpensive and viable option to treat fungal infections.

Chapter # 8: Lowers the Risk of Cancer

Cancer is a well-known class of disease that is characterized by abnormal growth of cells in any part of the body; cancer spreads throughout the body using the blood stream and as it progresses, chances of curing it get thinner. Cancer targets a single organ by dividing & growing itself resulting in the formation of tumors.

Colon cancer is a type of cancer that develops in the large intestine. It originates from small, benign tumors that overtime develop into life-threatening tissues. A study conducted by a team at the University Of Nova De Lisboa in Portugal showed that dichloromethane and ethanol extracts obtained from Thyme had a protective effect against colon tumors.

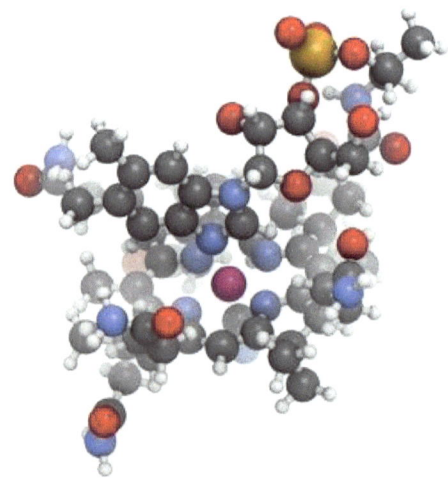

Thyme is also a very promising candidate for treatments of breast cancer. Oncologists at the Celal Bayar University in Turkey carried out tests to determine the effects of wild thyme on breast cancer activity. The team was looking out for programmed cell death (apoptosis) and changes in genes without tweaking with DNA (epigenetic events) in activated tumors. The extracts from thyme successfully initiated cell death in the tumors along with traces of gene changes that positively reflect onto the death of cancerous cells.

Thyme is also very rich in phenol content such as luteolin, apigenin, rosmarinic acid, eriodictyol and quercitin. Among these Luteolin has been recognized as the primary compound with anti-cancer properties. In a study that involved over 66,000 women, 1/5th of the women were kept on foods with high proportion of thyme. It was found that the risk of ovarian cancer dropped by 34% among these women, compared to the group that had no thyme consumption. In lab studies, luteolin decreased human ovarian cell development and lowered the amount of malign blood vessels formed due to cancer cells.

Chapter # 9: Alleviates High Blood Pressure

Many people relate blood pressure to as an obligatory entity that decides the rate at which our blood flows but in reality blood pressure is a force that drives blood through the body's whole circulatory system. Without this force, the two most basic provisions for life would get clogged up in our system:

i.   Oxygen

ii.   Nutrients

In addition to these two, blood pressure also delivers antibodies, insulin and white blood cells throughout the body. Blood travels through the body via a system of arteries & veins and just as reducing the width of a water pipe would increase the pressure of water that is output, the contraction of these arteries & veins has the same effect on blood. High blood pressure may be caused either due to the arteries getting narrowed or blocked.

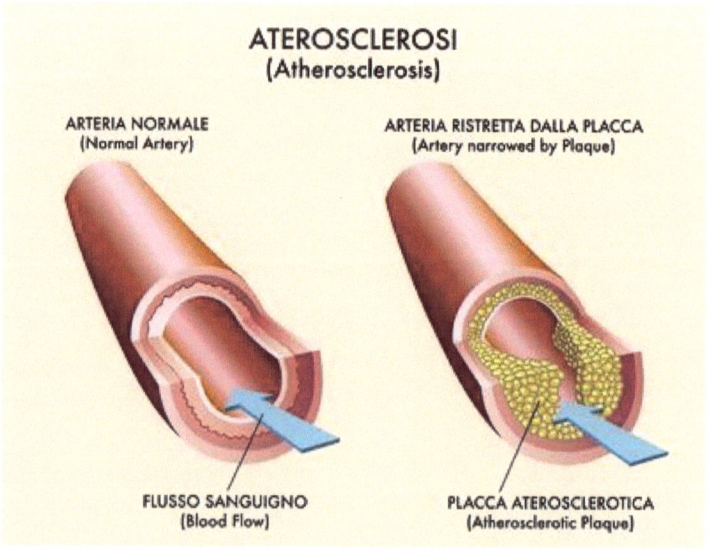

Researchers at the University Of Belgrade, Serbia were quite astonished of the fact that people belonging from the Mediterranean region didn't had a great risk of high blood pressure. A study involving an extract from thyme was carried out on laboratory rats to evaluate many blood pressure deciding factors like flavonoid contents, free radial scavenging and anti-oxidant capacity. The rats were divided into four groups, two of which received thyme extracts of different concentrations while the other two were kept on placebo diet. The results concluded that the group, which received the highest concentration of thyme extracts, had lowest oxidant activity and had a normalized blood pressure for the longest time, supporting the hypothesis that thyme lowers the chances of hypertension.

Chapter # 10: Food Preservative

As stated in the first health benefit, the oil of thyme can work against a variety of different bacteria & fungi. This specific property of thyme has been in use for thousands of years to preserve food items from microbial contamination. New research is showing that thyme not only protects from a microbial contamination but also decontaminates a previously tainted food item.

In one of these studies, published in the 2004, February issue of Food Microbiology, researchers revealed that the essential oil of thyme was able to purify a lettuce sample that was contaminated with an infectious organism known for triggering several intestinal diseases such as diarrhea; the organism is called shigella. In addition they were able to show that if lettuce was washed with solution containing just 1% thyme oil, the number of shigella bacteria dropped below the point of detection. This research is being used by scientists to develop food preservatives and anti-bacterial chemicals. It also wouldn't hurt you to incorporate thyme in more of your recipes that are uncooked, e.g. salads. Adding thyme to your vinaigrette will not only enhance its flavor but also heighten its nutritional benefits.

Another study carried out by Polish researchers, published in the November 2011 issue of Medicinal Chemistry, showed that thyme oil was effective in crushing bacteria that include Staphylococcus, Escherichia, Enterococcus and Pseudomonas genera. The thyme oils used were extracted from Thymus vulgaris and L. angustifolia. A total of 120 strains of bacteria were extracted from hospital environments and patients with infections in their respiratory, genitourinary & oral cavity tracts. The results showed that the oil extracted from thymes vulgaris was the most effective against all of the strains. Another study was carried out that compared the effectiveness of thyme oil with lavender oil against anti-biotic resistant bacterium strains. The results demonstrated that thyme was still the better oil against all types of strains when compared to lavender oil.

Studies surrounding the cellular benefits of thyme have shown that the essential oils of thyme can also be used as a potential anti-oxidant. Studies confined to laboratories reveal that the oil of thyme can protect and increase the proportion of healthy fats located in cell structures such as membranes. Specifically speaking, the amount of DHA, an omega-3 fatty acid present in kidneys, brain and heart cell membranes, was found to increase after the cells were injected with thyme oil supplements. Looking more closely at brain cells, researchers showed that the bodies of rats were able to reap maximum benefits when thyme was introduced early in their lifecycle; it was less effective when the rat had already aged.

The anti-oxidant effect of thyme is not limited to the body but can also be used in the food processing & storage industry. Lipid oxidation is considered a major problem during food storage and is known to cause loss in the stability, quality and nutritional value of food items. A study aimed at the preservation of sun flower oil with the help of thyme was carried out at the Institute of Food & Agricultural Biotechnology in Warsaw. Sunflower oil samples were kept in darkness at temperatures of 4 degree, 18 degree and 38 degree Celsius. The ethanol extract from thyme was added to the sunflower oil and a number of parameters including peroxide value, anisidine value and fatty acid contents were used to evaluate thyme's effectiveness. The final values of these parameters exhibited that thyme oil increased the lifetime of sunflower oil by acting as an anti-oxidant. The anti-oxidant property of thyme can be credited to the variety of flavonoids contained within thyme: apigenin, luteolin, naringenen and thymonin. These flavonoids combined with thyme's manganese content make it a high-standing item on the list of anti-oxidant herbs.

Chapter # 11: Treats Bronchitis

Bronchitis is an inflammatory, respiratory disease which involves the mucus membranes of the lungs' bronchial lining getting inflamed. As the inflamed membrane swells and becomes thicker in size, it narrows the airway in lungs and causes coughing accompanied by breathlessness and phlegm.

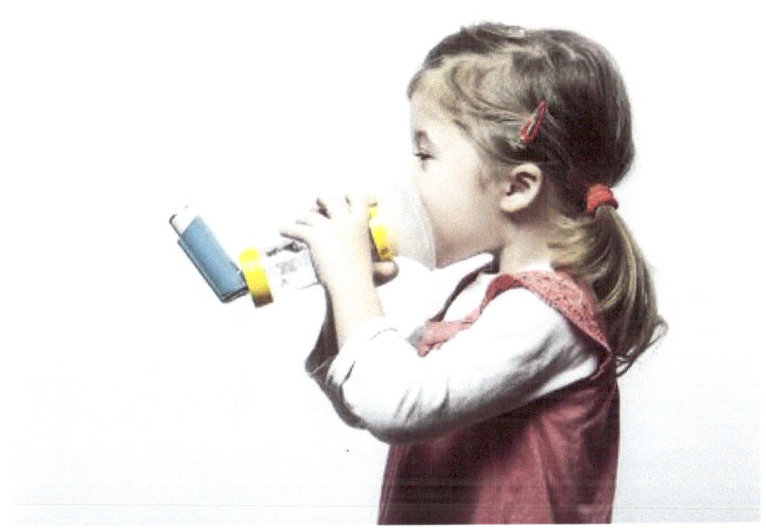

A research carried out by German scientists, published in the 2007 issue of Arzneimittelforschung evaluated the tolerability and efficacy of a fixed combination of primrose root with extracts from thyme plant on patients of cough and acute bronchitis. The results obtained from the combination were compared to placebo controlled treatment. A total of 361 patients who were suffering from acute bronchitis, with greater than 10 coughing episodes per day and a Bronchitis Severity Score of greater than 5 were randomly chosen and assigned to an eleven day treatment. 183 of the patients were each given a table of thyme-primose combination, 3 times a day while the rest stayed on a placebo treatment. The treatment was studied by counting the number of daily coughing fits and by the investigator himself. A 67.1% reduction in coughing fits was seen on the seventh and ninth day, before the end of the study. The group that was given a thyme-primose combination had a 50% reduction in coughing fits 2 days earlier than the placebo controlled group. Moreover, there was no safety risk and the treatment was well-tolerated by each patient.

The effectiveness of thyme oil was tested by researchers at the German Central Institute for Pharmaceutical Research. The researchers tracked the time taken by thyme oil to be absorbed into the bloodstream and the time it took to get fully broken down. The participants were given a 1.08 mg dose of thyme oil; the peak level of thyme in the bloodstream was found after 2 hours while the amount of oil kept decreasing up till 41 hours, after which it was no longer detected. This shows that thyme is quite quick to get injected into the body and stays in the bloodstream for a little less than 2 days which is a very respectable score for a natural medicine.

Chapter # 12: Kills the Tiger Mosquito

The tiger mosquito, known by its scientific name as Aedes albopictus is a native of the tropical & subtropical regions of Southeast Asia. Since the 1990s it has spread into other parts of the world and is notoriously known for transferring West Nile virus, St. Louis encephalitis, dengue fever and Yellow fever virus with it.

A team of researchers at the Chungbuk National University in South Korea carried out a study on the possible effects of oil of thyme in killing the larvae of tiger mosquitoes compared to other chemicals in different proportions. Their research was published in the September 2012 issue of the Journal of the American Mosquito Control. The following compounds were used:

i.	33% Gamma-Terpinene	vi	4.7% Mycrene
ii	29.9% Oil of Thyme	vii	4% Beta-Caryophyllene
iii	8.9% Beta-Bisabolene	viii	2.7% Alpha-Thujene
iv	8.3% Cymene	ix	1.3% Camphene
v	5% Alpha-Terpinene	x	1.2% Carvacrol
xi	1.1% Alpha-pinene		

Among all these candidates, thymol (the oil of thyme) proved to be the most effective one and exhibited 100% repellant activity against the female species.

Chapter # 13: Treats Yeast Infections

A yeast infection is a type of infectious disease that is characterized by irritation and itchiness in and around the area of the infection. The fungus Candida albicans is the most common cause of vaginal and mouth infections. Vaginal infections are often recurring and are popularly known as thrush. As many as 3 out of every 4 women experience this infection at some stage of their life. Researchers at the University of Turin, Italy studied the effect of the essential oil of thyme on Candida albicans, in an infected human specimen. The study was published in the 2012 issue of Planta Medica. The study showed that the essential oil at its minimal inhibitory concentration was able to significantly enhance the intracellular killing of albicans, in comparison to the non-essential oil treatment, which was pretty much ineffective against the infection.

Conclusion

A delicate looking herb with a powerful fragrance, thyme will definitely add a positive trend to your life. Thyme is readily available in the market and doesn't need too much attention if you come up to the decision to grow it. It is packed with nutritional and health promoting benefits of numerous minerals, which have been tapped into, for hundreds of year; the benefits can be as small as facial problems to as big as lung diseases. Moreover, it has a wonderful smell that makes it a perfect anti-septic. A lot of researches have been carried out to study the properties of thyme and all of them have shown that this herb is literally nature's aromatic blessing.

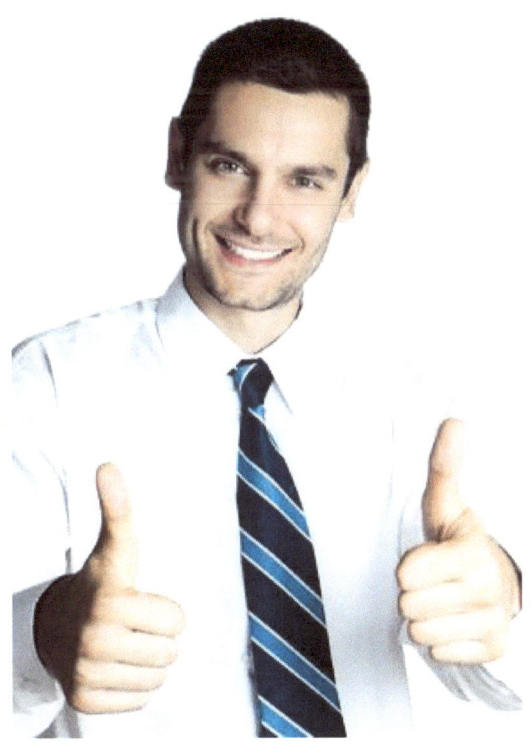

Everything about thyme, from its varieties to its benefits has been exemplified in this book. All you need to do is to simple follow it and add thyme to your daily diet for an enhanced, well-balanced and joyful life.

Author Bio

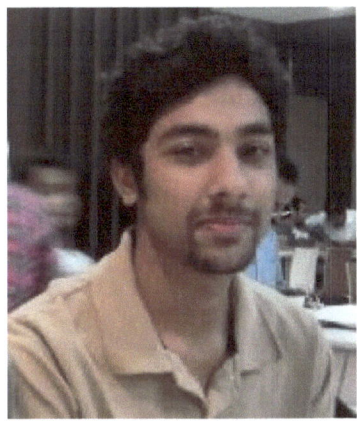

Muhammad Usman is a distinguished medical graduate of Allama iqbal medical college (AIMC). He is a professional writer who has been in the field for more than 4 years. During this time he has produced 10,000+ articles, blogs and eBooks on various niches related to diseases, health, fitness, nutrition and well-being. He is a regular contributor to several journals related to medicine and surgery. He is the editor of several journals and newspapers.

Check out some of the other JD-Biz Publishing books

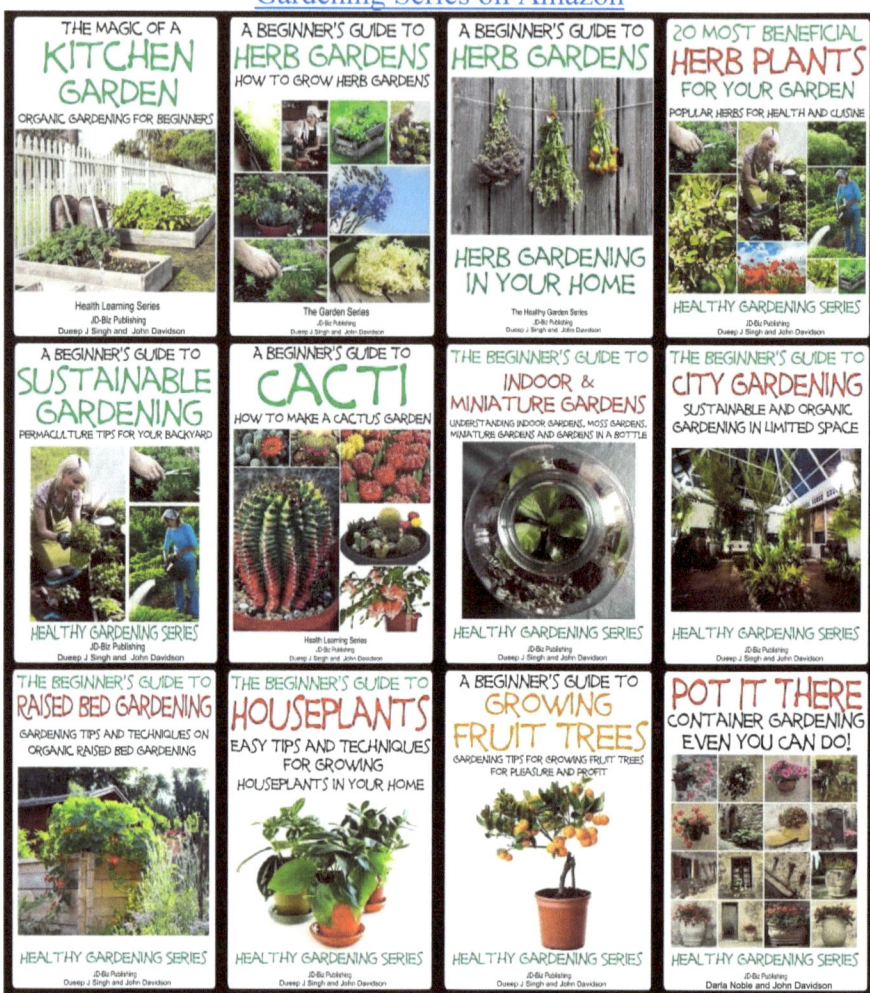

Health Learning Series

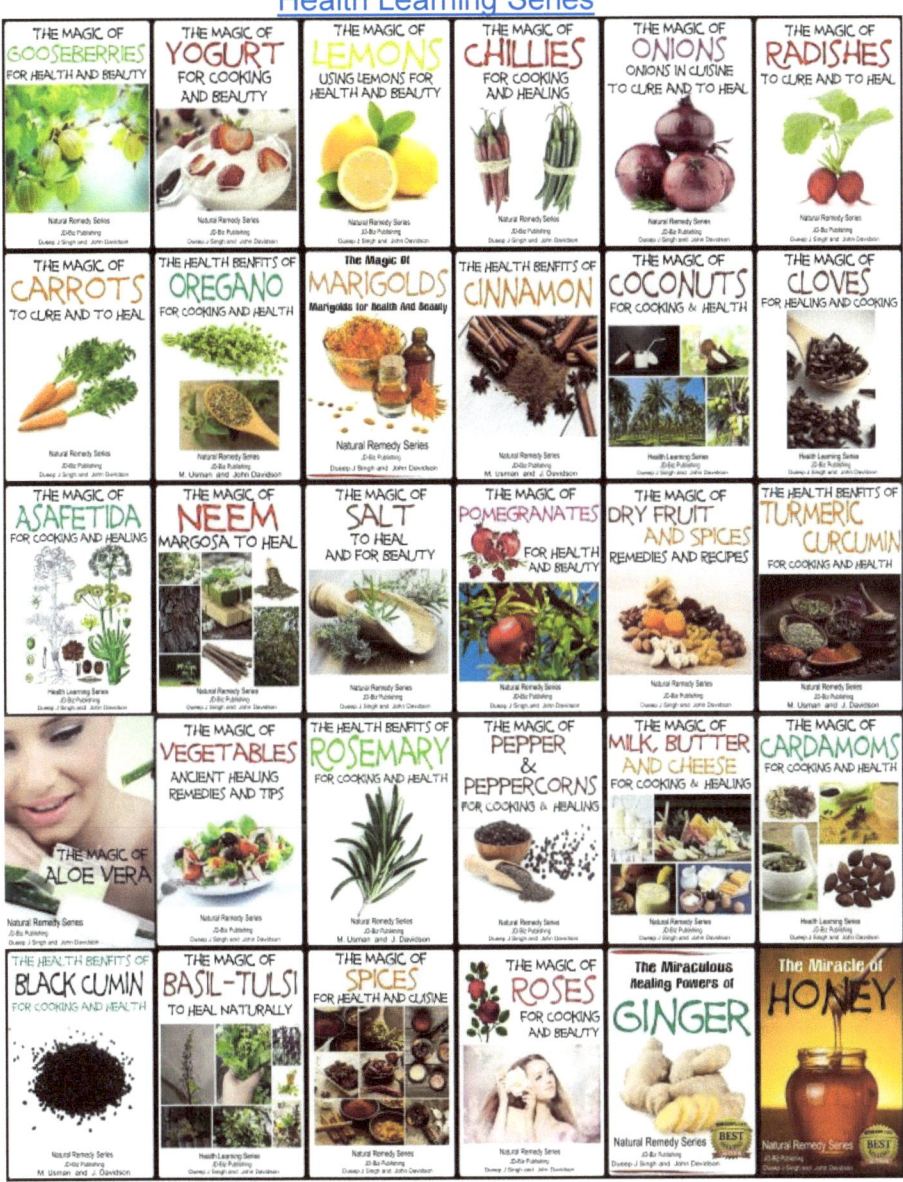

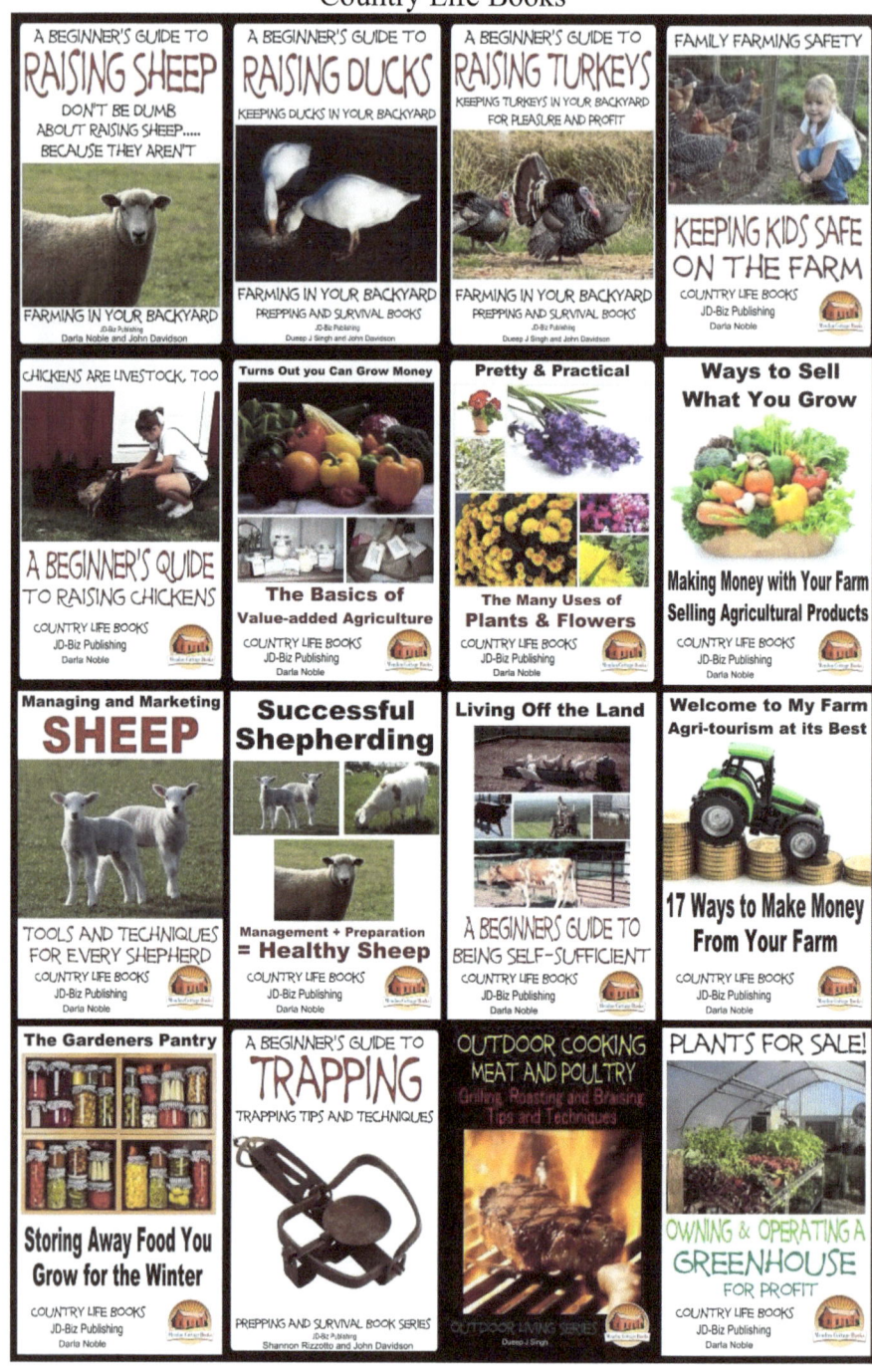

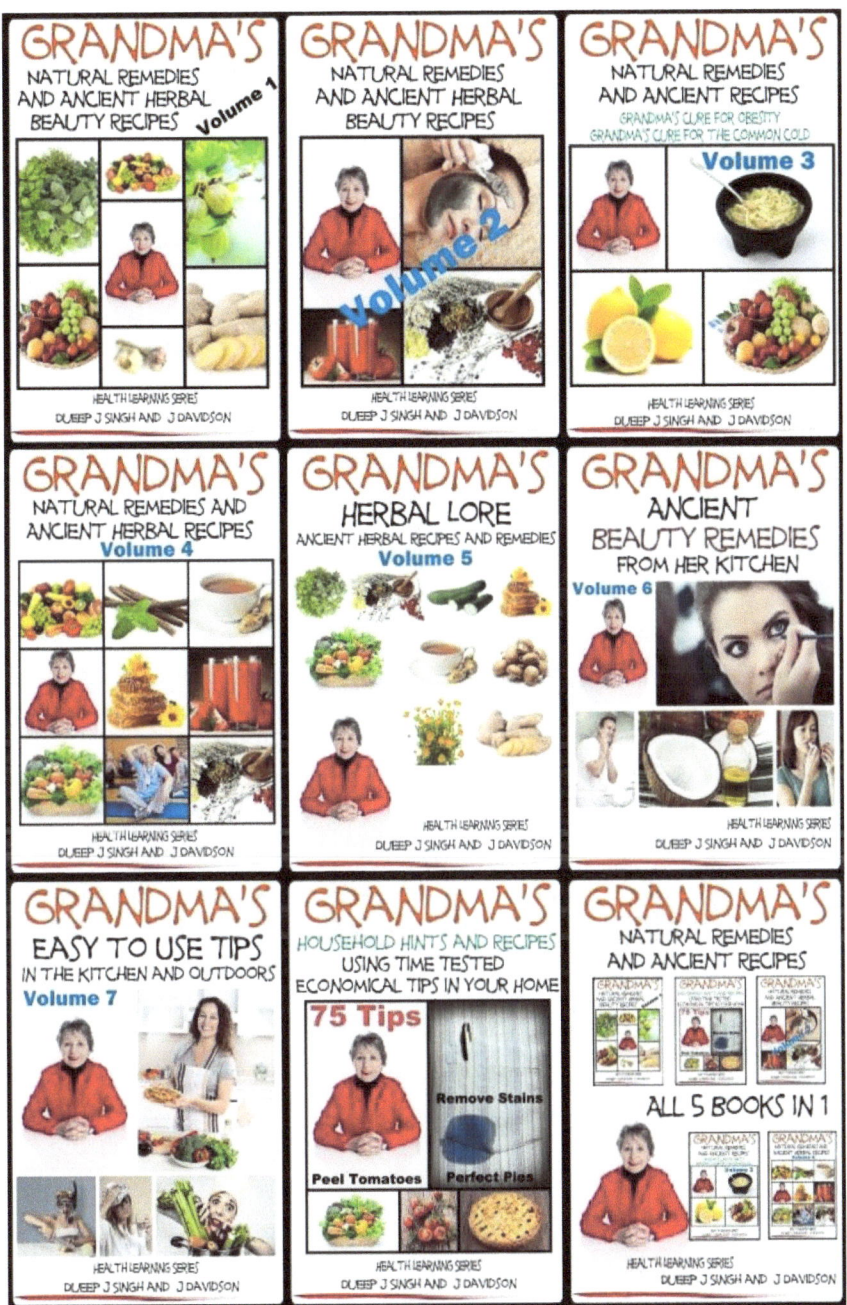

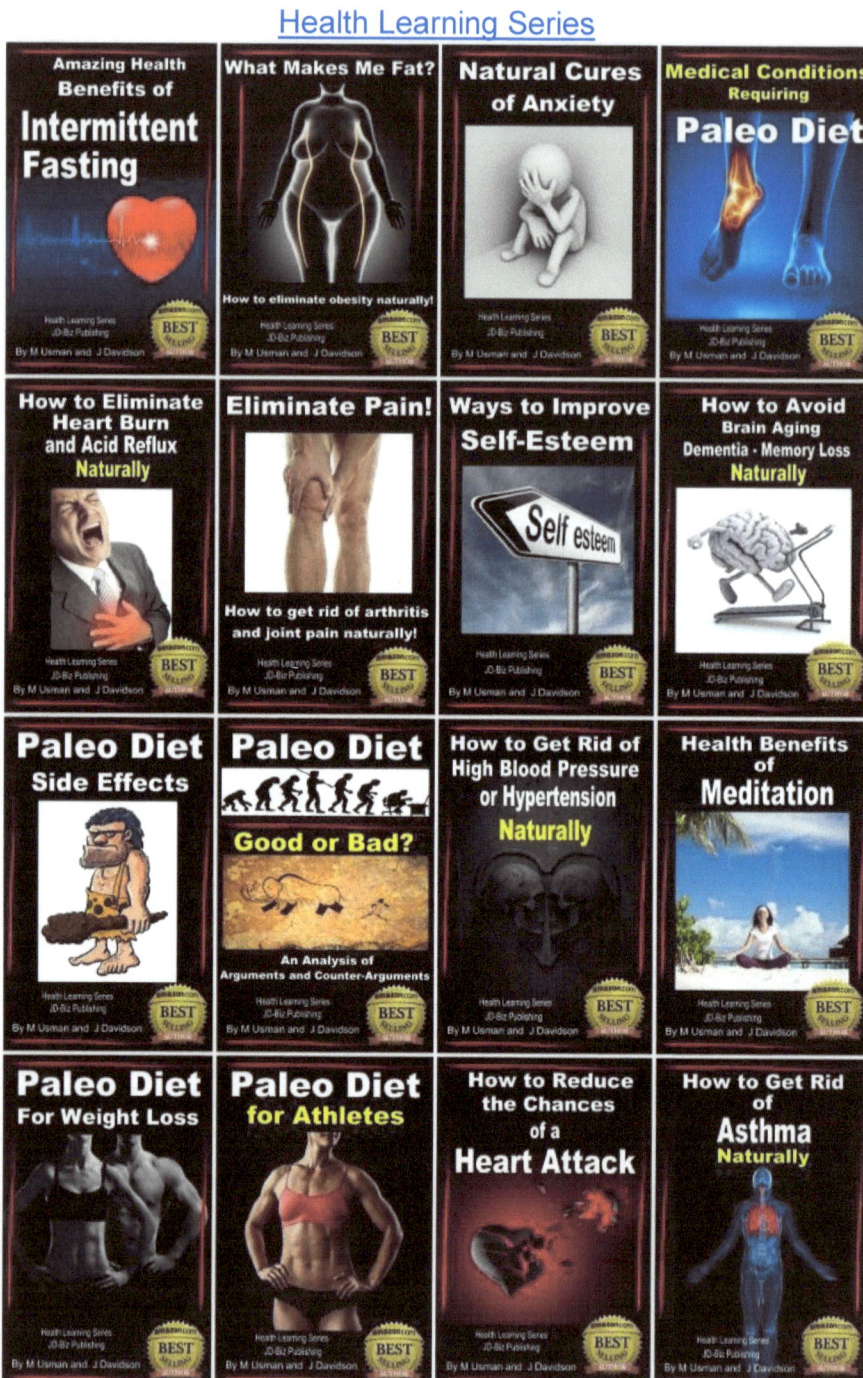

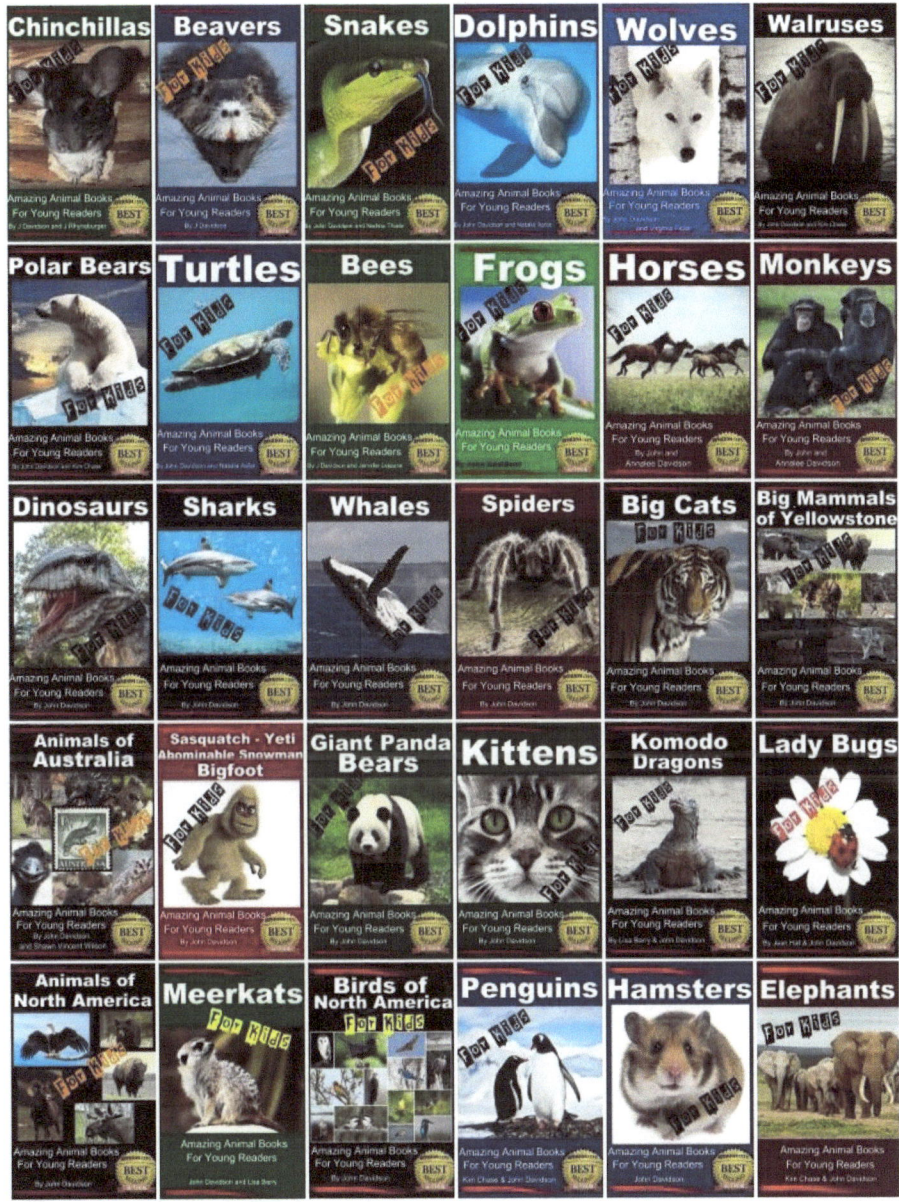

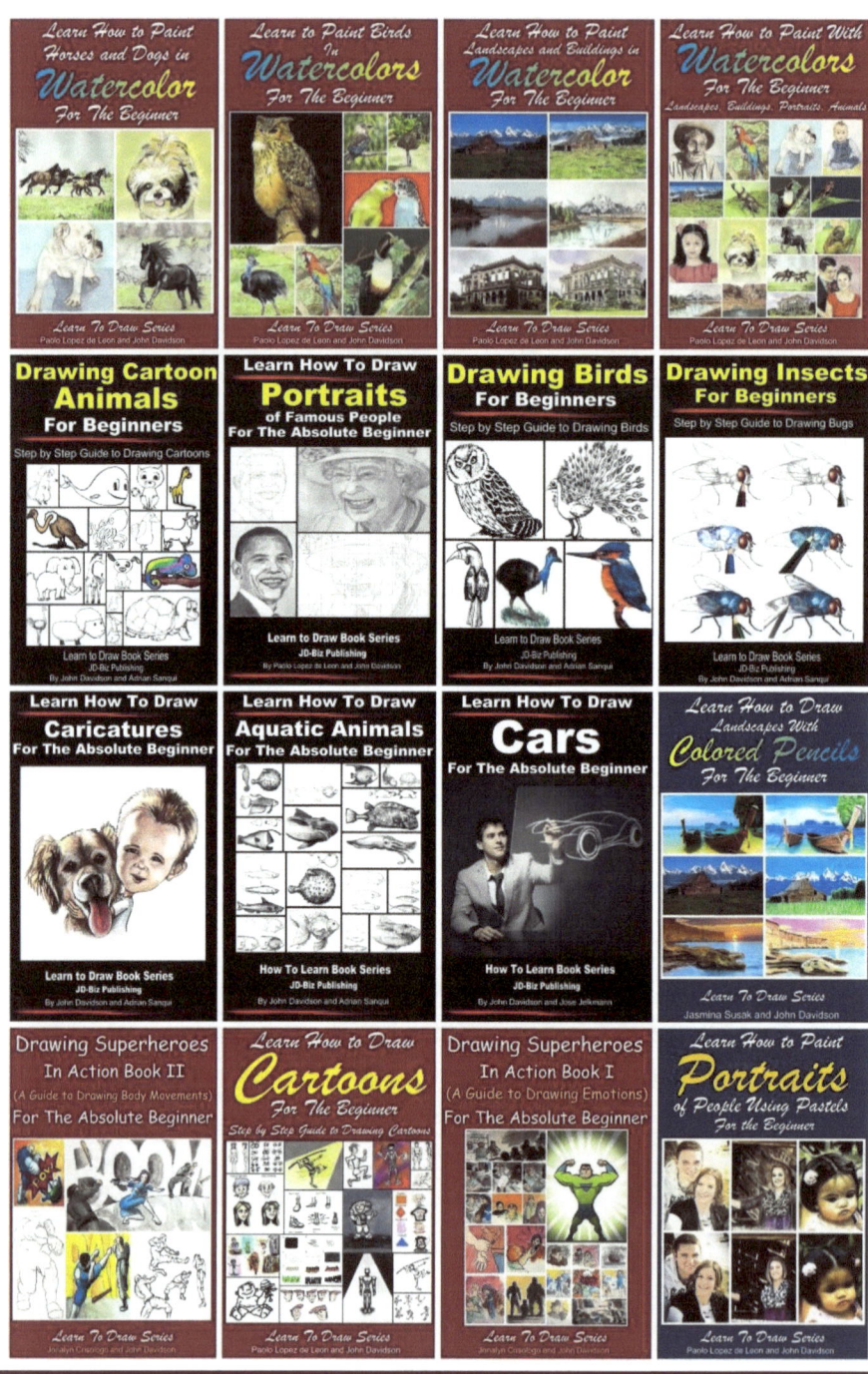

How to Build and Plan Books

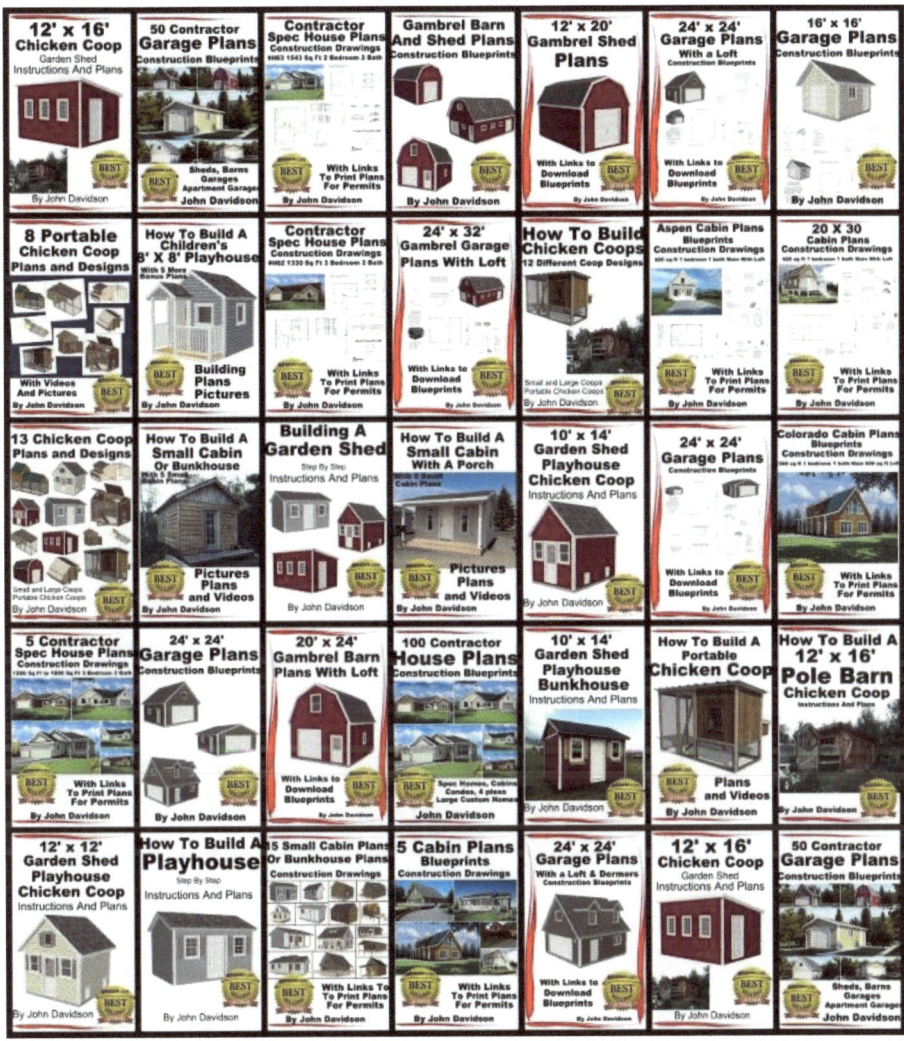

Entrepreneur Book Series

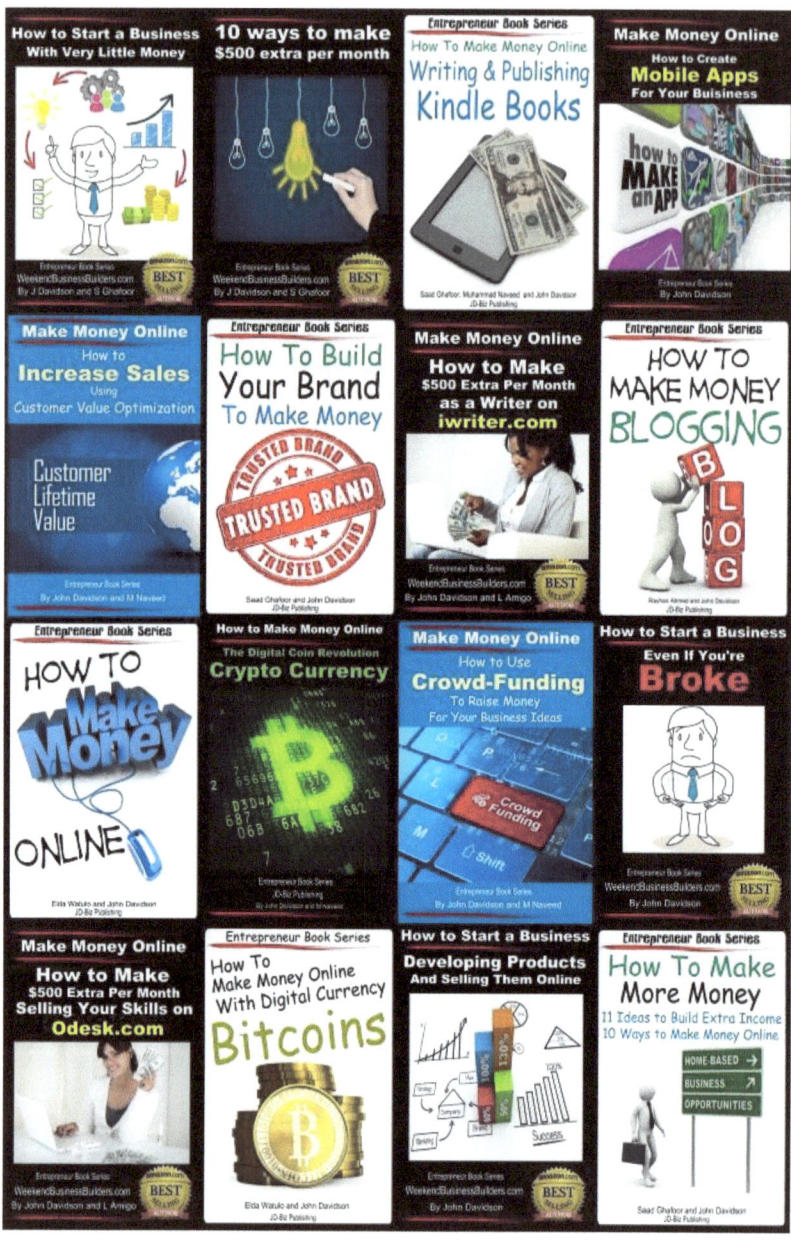

Our books are available at

1. Amazon.com
2. Barnes and Noble
3. Itunes
4. Kobo
5. Smashwords
6. Google Play Books

Download Free Books!

http://MendonCottageBooks.com

Publisher

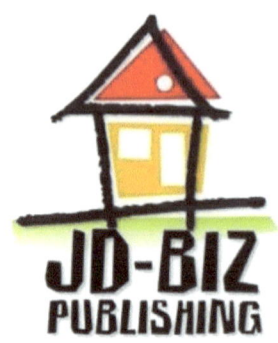

JD-Biz Corp

P O Box 374

Mendon, Utah 84325

http://www.jd-biz.com/

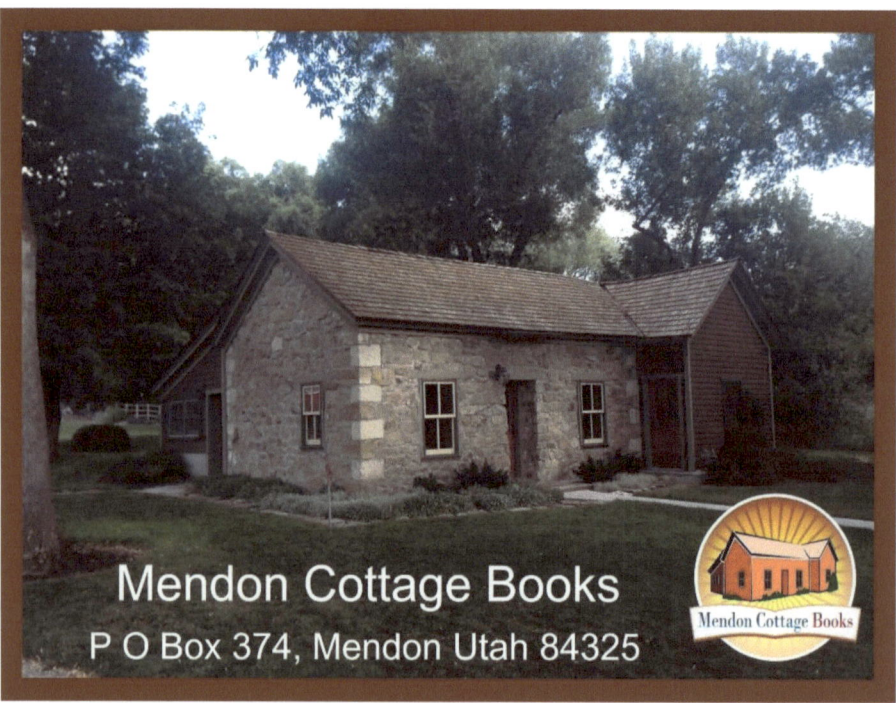

Mendon Cottage Books

P O Box 374, Mendon Utah 84325

www.ingramcontent.com/pod-product-compliance
Lightning Source LLC
Chambersburg PA
CBHW050837290526
45792CB00001B/430